T0146585

GO ASK DEBBIE

HEALTH AND FITNESS TIPS FROM A SEASONED EXPERT

DEBBIE CRALL

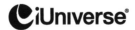

GO ASK DEBBIE
HEALTH AND FITNESS TIPS FROM A SEASONED EXPERT

iUniverse books may be ordered through booksellers or by contacting:

iUniverse
1663 Liberty Drive
Bloomington, IN 47403
www.iuniverse.com
1-800-Authors (1-800-288-4677)

Because of the dynamic nature of the Internet, any web addresses or links contained in this book may have changed since publication and may no longer be valid. The views expressed in this work are solely those of the author and do not necessarily reflect the views of the publisher, and the publisher hereby disclaims any responsibility for them.

Any people depicted in stock imagery provided by Thinkstock are models, and such images are being used for illustrative purposes only.
Certain stock imagery © Thinkstock.

ISBN: 978-1-5320-3792-4 (sc)
ISBN: 978-1-5320-3791-7 (e)

Library of Congress Control Number: 2018900556

Print information available on the last page.

iUniverse rev. date: 01/29/2018

CONTENTS

DEDICATION

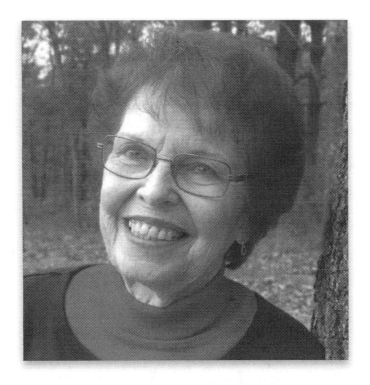

10-24-36 to 12-25-17

This book is dedicated to the most amazing woman in the world; my momma. Momma and I had a very close relationship and she had been a strong influence in my life. She taught me integrity, honesty and independence. Momma went to work every day and always had time to make us breakfast before school and dinner after she got home from a long day at work. She always made good healthy meals for us and rarely did I ever see soda or junk food in the house. She always got up and got dressed regardless of how she felt. The house was always organized and clean. And, yes, we had chores! Needless to say I came away with some good habits that were instilled in me as a child growing up.

Momma inspired me to write this book after she wrote and published her own book, "Dying For Answers".

I love and miss you so much Momma!

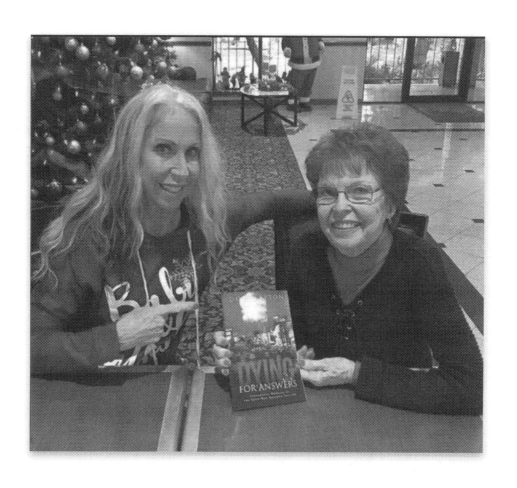

INTRODUCTION

This book is about health, fitness and nutrition. It is about the journey of a full time home-bound super mom with three small kids that needed a personal energy outlet besides watching soap operas, drinking Dr Pepper and smoking two packs of cigarettes a day. This is the story of a life reborn and purposed for living.

After over thirty-five years in the business of fitness, as a Certified Personal Trainer through National Academy of Sports Medicine, a seven-year veteran of competitive bodybuilding and a fitness model, I came to the conclusion that I have a desire to share with those interested in fitness and those wanting to embark on a fitness journey. I became motivated in 1981 when my Uncle Eric told me I was going downhill at 26 years old because I became winded running around the yard with the kids. I set out to do something about it.

I believe I have the right credentials to write this book based on my years of education, experience and research. I share my struggles, fears and setbacks along this path to wellness. My desire and motivation is that this book has the potential to impact your life whether you are a beginner or ready to take yourself to the next level. If you have a true desire to get healthy and attain an overall sense of wellness, this content will illuminate the path as you start your fitness journey. I learned everything the hard way and all I had was motivation and a deep desire to keep going. Hold on tight. Let me lead you forward to a new you.

ACKNOWLEDGEMENTS

Thank you mom and dad for great genetics. Your belief in me has made me be who I am today. I'm especially thankful to momma and my daughter Alynna for inspiring me to write this book.

Thank you to my most awesome kids Jeff, Alynna and Jon for allowing me to ever so gently place you on my shoulders for squats and lunges.

Special thanks to my amazing husband, Mike, for his endless support and love. I love you so much.

Thank you Keitha Story Stephenson for your guidance and coaching.

Thank you Doug and Jeannie Andrewski for your mentorship as I began my journey into the world of bodybuilding and Nutrition.

Thank you Samantha and Robert Reid for all of the training and guidance at Obstacle Warrior during my preparation for American Ninja Warrior.

Special thanks to Kelly Jimenez for your patience and confidence in me. I could not have made it as far as I did in competitive bodybuilding without your support!

CHAPTER 1

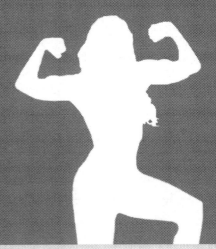

BIRTH OF A SUPER MOM

In 1981, I was visiting my Uncle Eric and Aunt Carol. We were just a bunch of relatives hanging out and having fun, listening to music and cooking out. I was running around outside with the kids and remember getting SO winded I couldn't keep up and it bothered me. I told my Uncle Eric that I was whooped. I told him that I wish I could keep up with them.

He said, "This is where you start to go downhill, Debbie. You're getting older so you had better be prepared to start going down hill."

"I'm only 26 years old," I replied.

"Yep, that's when it all starts. Better get ready," he explained. I drove off scratching my head. The thought had never occurred to me. But it started me thinking, 'Am I really getting old?' All the way home I took a closer look at my lifestyle and I did actually feel like I was melting into the couch everyday just watching soap operas, drinking Dr Pepper and smoking two packs of cigarettes a day. I woke up the next morning around 5:30am with no alarm. My first thought was 'this is it'. I'm not sleeping in to 9:30am anymore because I don't want to go downhill.' Apparently, I was still bothered by Eric's comment because it woke me up in the wee hours of the morning. I got up, went into the living room, turned on the television looking for an exercise show to start working out. There was *"Morning Stretch with Joanie Greggains"*. She was doing leg lifts in this cute little outfit talking about "no more road maps" on these thighs.

What's that, I said to myself? What is she talking about? I got up and went over to the mirror and it became very clear what she was talking about. There I stood looking at road maps on my thighs. I thought to myself, 'OH NO'! I've got those. I don't want that! So I got right back to work squeezing harder with every rep. The more I watched her, the more I was thinking, there is no way I can look like THAT, but I can at least follow her routine everyday and see what happens. I became very optimistic.

When her show ended another fitness show started. There in my living room was "Bess Motta with the Twenty-minute workout". She was another sassy, classy-looking, fitness gal in a cute little outfit doing leg lifts and a lot of other exercises I wanted to incorporate. Eventually, I invested in a cute little outfit to wear for workouts. It motivated me even more. New tights still keep me motivated me today. Every morning at 5:30am, I would hit the deck and work out with Joanie and Bess. They became my mentors and workouts were getting serious.

Within a few weeks working out with these rock stars, I began feeling more like super mom and ready for weight training. I didn't have any at the time and began looking around the house for anything heavy to lift - milk cartons, coffee table, kitchen table. My goal was to eventually lift my refrigerator but that never happened. I used the milk cartons for chest flies on the coffee table and lateral raises. It was my low-tech heavy workouts.

I was always fishing for something heavy to lift. I also had another great idea.

I could make this a family affair, teach my little ones about fitness and use them as my weight training sessions. I stacked one on my shoulders for squats and lunges doing fifteen repetitions. I would lift one kid up and down like an overhead press fifteen times… My children, Jeff, Alynna and Jon absolutely loved this journey of ours.

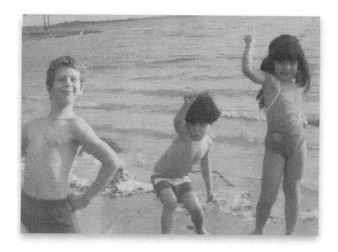

Grocery shopping became a fitness adventure as well. Before I knew it, my children were scouting the aisles for something heavy to lift. They began lifting milk cartons over their head and squatting ten-pound potato sacks. I began coaching by instructing, "Oh no baby, that's too heavy. Let's start with five pounds and work our way up to 10 pounds slowly." They loved being involved and had no problem including them on my journey that had become a family adventure.

Eventually, I bought a fitness book with detailed exercises and some light dumbbell workouts. That's when super mom became super serious. I remember how heavy the dumbbells were at first. I just knew I would get stronger if I did everything right and stayed consistent. After three weeks, I was ready to step up my game. For me, that was joining a gym. After calling around and getting some prices I discovered that I could not afford a gym membership. I was determined to find a way. In one phone call I asked the gym manager if aerobic instructors had to pay for membership. He said, "No". I replied, "Ok, I'll do that." He asked if I had any teaching experience. I guess working out at home for three weeks with Joanie and Bess just wasn't enough. I wondered how did you get experienced without "experience?" So I changed my approach. I just had one more call to make. It was at Elaine Powers Fitness Studio in Garland, Texas. The conversation went like this: Me: Hi, my name is Debbie. I'm wondering if you are hiring any aerobic instructors at this time?

Manager: Do you have any experience?

Me: Why, yes, I do. I've been trained by Joanie Greggains and Bess Motta. I've been working out with them for about three weeks.

Manager: REALLY?

Me: I laughed and told her that they were on my TV... I was in my living room. Then we both laughed.

Good way to break the ice, I guess because this is where I landed my first aerobic instructor job. I was so excited. I was all set to showcase my talents and eager to learn all I could about fitness. The manager at Elaine Powers Fitness Studio taught me an exercise routine that I was to lead the class through as I stood on a small stage. I remember being up there overlooking all these women, sweating to keep up. These women were serious. They were huffing and puffing and just grinding it out. I was amazed, because seriously, they were in better shape than I was at that time. This is where I learned about intensity because they pushed me. Then a two-Day Elaine Powers Certification Workshop came up in Dallas, Texas. It was free so I took advantage of the opportunity. I was out to learn all I could about fitness.

When we arrived at the venue, we were taught a basic routine. Our certification would be based on our completion of this routine at the conclusion of the workshop. I messed up on one part but still thought I did well. Afterwards, they called each of us over to let us know how we had been ranked. They called my name and I approached the bench and sat down. The judge informed me that she could not certify me. They felt I had not replicated the routine.

The next day I went right back to teaching, picking up where I left off. I had not learned anything in that workshop, with the exception of repeating a routine. By now, I had developed good training habits and ditched the old. I had taken control of my life. I had quit smoking and drinking Dr Pepper and lost track of what was going on with *All My Children, One Life To Live and General Hospital*. I was ok with that. I felt better and had more energy than I'd ever had. I was slowly but surely feeing more and more like a true SUPER MOM!!

CHAPTER 2

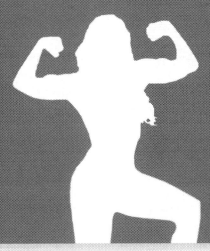

FAMILY MOVES TO TEXARKANA

In 1984, the family moved to Texarkana and by then I was totally infected with the fitness bug. I started making my calls to local fitness clubs to try and get back into teaching. I had gained experience and could not wait to become involved in the activity I loved. I couldn't wait to get back to teaching. I must have called this one gym one hundred times. The last time I called I remember saying, "What's the deal, pickle? Are you going hire me or not?

He laughed so hard and then replied, "Ok, come in and audition." I did and was immediately hired. I landed my second aerobic job at Jim Bottins Nautilus Plus and started teaching classes immediately. My class was held 5:30pm-6: 30pm Monday - Friday with day care. Right down my alley and with day care! This was a gym setting with a lot more people so I was a bit nervous. I managed to meet some amazing people who would inspire me throughout my life. My class became over crowded very quickly and I was honored the following year when they asked me to do an interview on my aerobic classes for a local newspaper. It cracked me up that they were trying to compare it to the movie, "Perfect", with John Travolta and Jamie Lee Curtis. If you've never seen the movie, Curtis' character is this very popular aerobic instructor in a high tech gym. In the movie, they had a sofa where members can congregate and get to know each other. It was equipped with tables and chairs in a bar setting, (I'm not talking about barbell either) I'm talking about a bar that served alcohol.

Jim Bottins, Nautilus Plus was nothing in comparison but I certainly enjoyed the interview. I remember the interviewer asking me if I can compare my gym to the movie "Perfect" and I replied, No way, I believe people are here strictly here to get in shape and to workout. They don't serve beer there. The article said I was the most demanding and popular aerobic instructor at the gym. I was very honored. It helps to love what you do. A few months later I was asked by the same gym to do a hot tub commercial. Of course, I said yes. I was ready but was hesitant to strut out in a bathing suit but I was able to do this one-minute commercial that took about five takes with no problems at all.

I remember one evening during one of my classes a cameraman came into my aerobics class and was photographing and video taping my feet. Just my feet. I was wearing my bright yellow Reebok© shoes bouncing around. When I asked what he was doing, he said that is a study on Reebok© shoes. And, that was it.

Aerobic Competitions Began

In 1985, I was informed about an upcoming aerobic competition. The other Instructors and I decided to enter. We had a blast. We all worked really hard on our routines which had to include four sit-ups, four jumping jacks, four high leg kicks and four push-ups. I made up a routine and ended up winning the whole thing. I took home $100.00 and two trophies. That was the first and last time I ever won any money in competitions.

I honestly didn't think I was as polished as the other girls but I remember how much fun it was and I was happy that the judges liked me. My family and half of my aerobic class were there, cheering me on. They were all wearing shirts that said, "Debbie's Gang" printed on the front. I had a great support team. I later went on to compete in the Arkansas State Aerobic Competition in Hot Springs, Ark in 1985 where I finished in 4th. I competed a couple more times and then stopped.

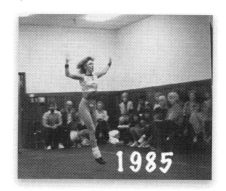

CHAPTER 3

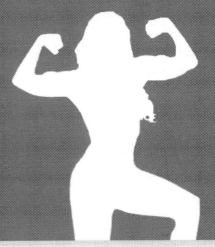

FAMILY MOVES TO WISCONSIN

In 1986, the family moved to Wisconsin. I was heartbroken to be leaving behind all the people that had become close friends. I remember receiving one particular phone call from a lady who called crying because I was leaving. It literally broke my heart. She said she lost sixty pounds in my class. I had no idea. This made a huge impact with me because it wasn't until then that I realized my calling. I am called to help people get healthy. I'm here to motivate and inspire others and to help them change bad habits and live a healthy productive life. How rewarding.

I landed another aerobic instructor job in Wisconsin Rapids, Wisconsin and loved it there. Here's a picture of me in 1986 after an aerobics class. I searched around for aerobic contests but couldn't find any nearby. That was okay with me because I was obviously led to do something else. BODYBUILDING! Everything happens for a reason and at the right time.

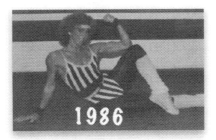

Bodybuilding World Here I Come

My husband at the time, Kelly, had his doubts at first about my competing but eventually ended up being very supportive. He was on the road during the week and home only on the weekends so what's a woman to do? So, I got a hobby! It was bodybuilding.

I told Kelly one day I was going to enter a bodybuilding competition and that people at the gym were encouraging me to enter the 1986 Stevens Point Bodybuilding Competition coming up. Kelly and I both thought at the time that everyone who did these shows were on steroids and no way I could look like that but I still wanted to give competition a try. I had never even been to a bodybuilding show. I have seen a few bodybuilding women training in the gym but never considered myself one of those women.

What do they do on stage in that bikini? I actually thought that they were a little too muscular and vascular for my liking but was curious as to how I would do, nonetheless.

Prejudging was the morning before the night show and each contestant had to do a 90 second routine with no music and just them posing on stage highlighting their strengths. I had no idea what mine were so, of course, I had to wing it and just watch the other girls to see what they were doing. Then, it was my turn. I remember having loads of fun, bouncing around and flexing my muscles like I knew what I was doing.

Next came the line up and some mandatory poses. The judges called out a front double bicep. I didn't get that memo. Are we supposed to have two biceps in one arm? I was clueless but my peripheral vision helped me a little bit. I was shuffled around a lot. They moved me far right, then far left, then to the middle. What's going on here, I thought. Why are they moving me around like this? Comparison is what was going on. The judges move you around to compare you side-by-side to another similar body type. The word was, back then, that prejudging apparently was where the competition was won or lost. After morning prejudging, I loaded up the kids, went home, rested up and we came back at night for the show and awards. We had a 90 second routine we did to our selected music. My song was "I sweat" and it was an upbeat and bouncy routine. This was fun and I remember absolutely loving the stage. I ended up winning my first competition! Not just my weight class but also the competition overall.

Kelly wasn't able to attend my first competition but my kids were all there on the front row yelling; GO MOM! I came home, called Kelly and told him I won! We were actually both very surprised. He asked, how did you do that? I replied, I don't know. I just know it was a lot of fun and I want to do it again.

We both learned very quickly that there were special tools that the judges were looking for, and yes, size was one of them but so was symmetry, proportion, posing, stage presence, tanning, routine and comparison. Then, it was GAME ON! Wow! OH, What a night!

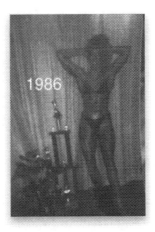

I went on to compete in another show that was held in Madison, Wisconsin, a couple of weeks later in which I won first in my class and first overall yet again. I did another competition, then another one, then another back to back. I was definitely on a roll winning and placing high so I kept the fun going.

I did have meltdowns after each show though. I remember just crying my eyes out because I didn't know what I wanted to do next. I believe this is why I competed for so many years. I was having fun and eventually it would lead to something else, a new adventure. I just didn't know what. I became an avid reader of <u>Muscle and Fitness</u> and Rachel McLish instantly became my inspiration. She was the first Ms. Olympia bodybuilder. She was small, muscular and very feminine. Pro-bodybuilder Cory Everson stormed the scene with an even more muscular physique but still very feminine.

These were two of my favorite women bodybuilders and I looked forward to reading about them every month. There were not many resources back then. All I had to learn from was <u>Muscle and Fitness</u> and <u>Flex Magazine</u>. I read everything I could get my hands on that pertained to health and fitness. Eventually I would become featured in *Flex Magazine*. That's another piece of memorabilia I would love to get my hands on. I remember thinking that I wish I had a personal trainer. It seemed like everybody had a personal trainer except for me. I had no choice but to teach myself. I felt like I needed someone who had already been through this. A pro. Someone like Cory Everson or Rachel McLish, but no such luck.

As a result, I became self-taught. Eventually, I met fairly knowledgeable people that I could go to with questions, but I wasn't receiving professional guidance like I wanted. I was infected with the fitness bug so I was focused, driven and motivated and apparently that's all it took, because before you knew it…. I not only had one Trainer - BUT TWO!

Meet My New Trainers

The mirror and the camera became my trusty Trainers. I started practicing in front of a full length mirror everyday and my kids took progression pictures for Comparison. These two things helped me determine what I needed to focus on. I evaluated myself again, reading everything I could get my hands on regarding fitness and nutrition. If I saw that my butt needed firming up and my back and shoulders needed to widen to get that symmetry I knew exactly what to do to make that happen.

My posing sessions became my favorite part of contest prep and I was actually getting pretty good at it. In 1988, I won "Best Poser Award" at one competition in Appleton, Wisconsin. There were 25 competitors.

The mirror and camera helped me so much. I was becoming a little ham in front of these two. I have actually been a little show off all my life, which is probably why my daddy nicknamed me Prissy.

It was shortly after winning the show in Madison that the owner of the gym where I worked out told me about a Personal Trainer, Doug Andrewski and his wife Jeannie, both big time competitors of the sport and extremely knowledgeable. I made the call and Doug and Jeannie were so approachable to answer any questions I had regarding the competitions, nutrition, and posing. They became great mentors and I learned so much. I would contact Doug before and after my shows to get feedback. I was so grateful for their leadership and experience. He had been training three other competitors at the gym. I personally could not afford his services so I continued my journey into the bodybuilding world turning to my trusty mirror and my camera to help guide me plus communicating with Doug and Jeannie via phone calls.

Nutrition became the next biggest and most important focus I would seek to understand. I recognized that this was half the battle if I were to take this to the next level. Doug and Jeannie suggested that I try different "peaking" techniques. One being carb loading (carb deplete then carb load) not sure how many grams of carbs I took in but it went something like this: Day 1. Cut back 50 grams of carbs. Day 2. Cut back another 50 gms of carbs. I continued this each day until I reached ketosis. I had bought ketosis sticks and stayed right on top of it checking it frequently. Then, at the right time, I would gradually start adding back in my carbs up to the night of the show, which averaged out to be 500gm that last day I think. It was amazing to see the changes when I actually peaked. I didn't always peak at the right time, but that's just the way it was. I was so ripped it didn't matter all that much. Another technique was sodium loading. I'm not sure exactly how that went but I only tried it once and will never ever do it again. I think that was the competition where I placed 3rd. I looked horrible and very water logged.

So after logging and testing my body, I recorded exactly how I felt after eating, along with detailed notes about how I looked and felt. Did I suddenly get a headache? Was I bloated? Was I tired? I did this for almost two years. This took me a while to figure out but still I ended up hitting my peak most of the time and when I did, I was on point - Full and tight everywhere. I learned a vast amount and I thank Doug and Jeannie for sharing their knowledge and expertise.

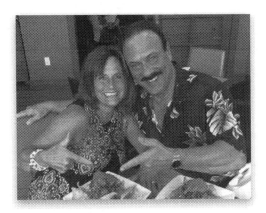

Off to the Nationals

By now I had won several National Qualifiers so just for the heck of it, in 1989, I flew out to Las Vegas and competed at the NPC North American Nationals Championships. What a blessing to be in the presence of all these pros. When I started working out, I had no aspirations of being Ms Olympia or enter a National show. I was basically just having fun and seeing how far I could take this without having a major commitment. I still had three small children at home and they were my priority.

There I was in Las Vegas at the Nationals standing in line at the weigh in and in front of me stood Linda Murray. The girl's body was dense with a lot of muscle. She had this tiny waist, flaring quads and shoulders, a huge back and she had this unique shape to her. I remember reading about her in the muscle magazines and there I was standing behind her at the Nationals. I introduced myself and told her that I thought she was the next Ms Olympia! She laughed and said, "Girl, I hope so!!" AND SHE WAS!

I had always had this fear of making my weight class, which was 114-125 for middleweights. While I competed in all weight levels, middleweight, lightweight and heavyweight, I looked my best as a middleweight but the upper end of it. I stepped on the scale and it was 126! Total dévastation! How could I be one pound over? I had no choice but to compete with the heavyweights. I hadn't been training as long as the rest of the girls so my density wasn't there to compete with the big gals. I consoled myself by thinking, 'Just a couple more years and I'll be back.' But I never went back and I've always believed everything happens for a reason AND at the right time. I did however; deserve to be there. I had earned my spot and it was an honor to just be surrounded by these athletes whether you brought home a trophy or not.

Chapter 4

FAMILY MOVES BACK TO TEXARKANA

In 1991, the family moved back to Texarkana and I went to work for a new gym in town. I started teaching step class and body sculpting classes. I also did personal training on the side.

In 1993, I had one more show before hanging up my posing suit. It was the Arkansas State Bodybuilding Competition in Little Rock, Arkansas. A local gym called me asking me to do a photo/video shoot the day before the competition. I explained to them that I had been carbing up for a show so to overexert at that point would not be a good idea. I agreed to do the photo shoot. I was actually supposed to be resting. I was on point and ready to step on stage. When I got there, they asked me to do a few dumbbell curls and in order for me to do that I had to lift dumbbells. I got a little carried away enjoying myself and the cameras everywhere (remember, I'm a ham) and I ended up doing a little too much. I wanted a good photo/video shoot, so naturally I had an amazing workout during this time. The next day, I woke up and had flattened out. I panicked. I knew better. Shame on me.

BUT, I WIN!! FIRST IN MY CLASS AND FIRST OVERALL! OH, WHAT A NIGHT!

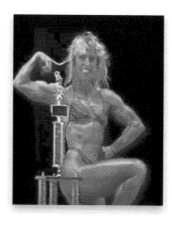

My family was on the front row screaming and the crowd was going crazy. I just stood there with tears rolling down my face. It was a very emotional night for me. I knew this was my last show and here I was crying again. I cried all the way home. I hung up my posing suit that night in June 1993 with 17 titles under my Champion Valeo belt. I was ready for my next adventure whatever that was to be.

After 7 years of competitive bodybuilding, it takes a toll on your body and I just felt it was time to move on. I had a blast and took my kids to every single competition except the Nationals. I have so many fun memories and I still hear their little voices "GO MOM" while sitting there on their front row. I have a ton of good memories. It is funny how during all these years as I posed on stage, I pictured myself posing with a mirror in front of me! It was an easy process for me and each time was a BLAST! The audience never scared me. I pranced out like, 'Woo Hoo, check me out.'

In 1995, I went to college to take an EMT course. I graduated and worked on the ambulance on call for a short while and continued to train hard. I did compete one more time. In 2016, just for the heck of it, I placed in the top 5 in the 45 and over at a local NPC show in Dallas. I was 60 years old.

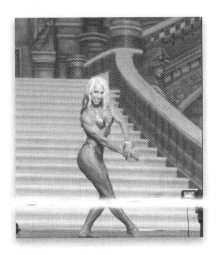

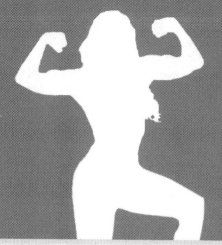

CHAPTER 5

SYMMETRY SIZE AND PROPORTIONS

Competitions can be a lot of fun but I'll have to admit they are just plain confusing. It's pretty much apples to oranges and those judges have their work cut out. Believe me, if you had a different set of judges, your placing would be different every time. It's just a judgment call because every one of those gals are in shape. Everyone is judged based on shape, size, stage presentation, but most of all, symmetry and proportion, presentation and a lot of hope that the judges would like you. How do you size up to the other gals? How do you present yourself?

Symmetry

Here is a picture of me two days before a show back in 1991. I weighed 124 lbs.

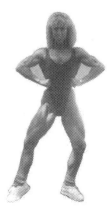

It took me 10 years to acquire this symmetry and progress came slowly. Genetics play a huge role as well. I have been very blessed. Thanks, mom and dad.

Sometimes it takes a skilled eye to actually see and compare you to others in a line up.

All I knew was that I was winning and placing high and having fun. I was enjoying this little hobby of mine so I continued. It was an expensive hobby but it was nothing compared to what competitions cost today.

The Cost of Competitions Back in My Days of Competing

Back in my competition days, I paid $35.00 for my posing suit. I can tell you I like the older suits better because they covered a lot more than what is covered today. Entry fees were $25.00. I did my own hair and make up. My tanning solution called, Dyoderm, that cost $15.00, came in a bottle and I tanned myself 3-4 days before. I prepared my own music on a cassette tape, gave it to the sound guy and that was it. It was still expensive. There were also hotel rooms, food, amino acids and a lot of food! It was just a rewarding hobby in which I thrived.

The Cost of Competitions Today

Before you begin reading this next section please understand that I'm not putting competitions down. All I am saying here is that it is vastly different today than in the days I competed as a bodybuilder, cost wise and categories. Today you might pay anywhere from $400.00 - $2000.00 and up for a posing suit alone. Shoes may or may not be worn depending on what category you enter but they run from $100.00 - $200.00 and up. Hair and make up costs a pretty penny too, but, if you know someone who could do yours, you will save a ton of money. My daughter, Alynna, did my make up for my last competition in 2016 and I was thrilled with it. She and Lana also helped with my hair. There is also the expense of tanning, travel and accommodations.

You'll be lucky to walk away with a trophy. The categories these days are plentiful. Fitness, Bikini, Figure, Physique, Bodybuilding, the list goes on...I tried judging these things at one point and it was like watching paint dry. Watching two hundred bikini competitors grace the stage, then figure category, physique, bodybuilding and God knows what else, not to mention the fact, competitors can enter as many categories as they wanted can get tiring. This is not only confusing to the audience but to the competitors as well. It can be extremely stressful and draining on a judge as well as on the competition. I understand people enter competitions for different reasons but I believe that everyone has a desire to win! Just keep this in mind: You are already a winner when you grace that stage after weeks of prepping yourself whether you bring home a trophy or not. Not everyone has the genetics to take it to a higher level like grabbing that Ms Olympia title or getting endorsements. Whatever you do, have fun doing it and above all, do it naturally and without drugs. Nothing is worth pumping your body with steroids and harmful supplements. My advice would be for you to train and hang with natural athletes. Be homemade. The beautiful thing about bodybuilding is you can change up your workout anytime and start training in the maintenance phase when you reach a point where you want to be. Getting there is all the fun but definitely attainable.

CHAPTER 6

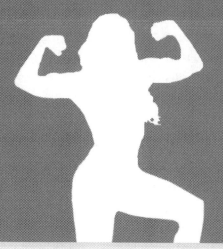

BUSTING THE MYTHS

Myth #1

You must spend three hours in the gym every day to get good results.

Truth

You can get serious results in 30-45 minutes per day if your workout is planned accordingly. Three times a week is sufficient. When you combine cardio and strength training together with proper nutrition and consistency, great things take place. Take out the chitchat and get serious.

Myth #2

You must do a lot of cardio to lose body fat.

Truth

Don't rely on cardio equipment as your only means of cardio. Try a Tabata workouts which consists of twenty seconds of exercise followed by a rest period of ten seconds for eight rounds. HIIT workouts are good as well. (High Intensity Interval Training) By this I mean pick about 5-10 exercises and do thirty seconds on each one back to back going from one exercise to the next with little or no rest. My favorite is, Jump Pulls, Wall Balls, Squat Jumps, Jump Rope, Push Ups.

You want to incorporate weight-bearing exercises into your routine. Basic compound moves that involve multi-joint movements like squats, lunges, and push-ups for a major calorie burn.

FYI - Cardio after a weight training session burns more calories verses before a workout. If you really want to get serious do high intensity weight training early in the morning. You will burn more calories and keep that metabolism revved up throughout the day.

Myth #3

Weight training builds bulky muscles in women

Truth

This depends on what "type" of training you are doing and the calories you are consuming. Your muscle tissue is actively burning fat. Weight training actually creates bone density and tightness in the muscle. If you use more weight in perfect form and get better results, you will spend less time working out. Don't be afraid. Once people actually start working out with weights, two things happen.

1. They begin to see changes in their bodies and like what they see.
2. They realize just how hard you have to work and how difficult it is to develop a really significant amount of extra muscle mass.

Myth #4

Free weights are dangerous

Truth

Free weights are safe when used properly. Yes, they are challenging because they involve more muscles groups to assist you in a single exercise. The more muscles you use when you workout, the more calories you will burn, and the less time you will need to workout. Just be intense.

Myth #5

Doing more abdominal exercises will burn fat around the waistline

Truth

There is no effective way to spot reduce anywhere on your body. Most people burn calories all over the body. When we store them, most people typically store them in one specific place on the body, not all over. Which doesn't make much sense to me scientifically. I mean, if fat metabolizes evenly, why do we store it in one spot. If you are one of those who store it all over, you are blessed. The best way to get a thin waistline is proper exercise and clean eating, not just sit-ups and abdominal exercises. I get this question often while pinching their belly: How do I get rid of this?

Abdominals are made in the kitchen, ya'll.

Myth #6

You must weigh on the scale every day to keep in check

Truth

Don't tell me…. You've weighed at least twice today, right? If you did, were you happy with what the numbers said? When are you going to stop beating yourself up over stupid numbers? Seriously! Stop it! The human body is a complex piece of machinery. I've been studying/ researching it half my life. There are a lot of things going in, coming out, transforming and dissolving all the time.

As a result, your weight can fluctuate wildly over the course of a 24-48 hour period. Your weight can go up 5-8 pounds depending on what you ate, how much water you drank, how much water you are retaining based on the amount of salt you've had, (oh, hey sodium), what time of day you weigh and many other factors. Therefore, your weight will be different every time you step on that scale.

Here are some better ways to measure your fitness progressions: the mirror, the ways your clothes fit, strength gains, pinch test. It makes me laugh and frustrates me at the same time to see people hop on the scale only to have a meltdown because they gained a pound, or lost only two. If they gained a pound, I tell them to go have a bowel movement. That'll help tip the numbers.

Unless you are training for a specific weight class event or you are morbidly obese and your doctor tracks your weight, toss the scale! It's a poor way to chart your progress. Body composition (the amount of fat and muscle in your body) is more important tool for tracking your progress versus the number on the scale.

Cutting calories and eating the wrong types of food can actually slow down your metabolism and reduce muscle mass. When this happens, your metabolism will stop burning calories and slow down, which creates the perfect environment for your body to become more efficient at storing fat rather than burning it. In most cases, you will lose weight, but predominately muscle weight, which results in you being a thinner person with a higher percentage of fat. I call that FAT THIN! Remember, MUSCLE BURNS CALORIES. SIMPLE OVERVIEW: Stay off the scale. It will make you cry.

CHAPTER 7

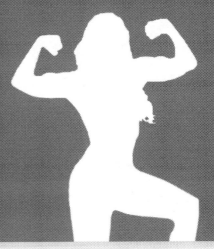

MUSCLE SORENESS, RECOVERY & OVERTRAINING

Sometimes muscle soreness happens and sometimes it doesn't. Not to worry. Muscle soreness is not a prerequisite and in no way an indication of whether the workout was good or not. I have also heard people say they don't exercise because they hate being sore. I honestly don't know how anyone can avoid muscle soreness at some point and time from their training.

DOMS, Delayed Onset Muscle Soreness, usually comes with a 24-48 hour period after the workout. If you experience muscle soreness, address the issue by gentle walking or massage. Remember, whether you can walk the next day after a leg workout or not, doesn't mean you've wasted your time or didn't get a good workout. Everyone's body reacts differently.

It's funny how some of my clients actually think that it was me that kicked their butt. I made them sore. Nope, It's all on them. I designed the workout and they pick their own intensity based on how they feel that particular day. I simply lie out the plan of action and make sure they executed the moves properly along with a few words of encouragement. It's their workout and they are responsible for their own intensity.

If you absolutely hate muscle soreness, go easier on your intensity, take more time to rest in between your sets, drink more water to stay hydrated, make sure you are properly fueled up before the workout and you get in your protein/carb meal within 2 hours after. Get some quality rest. Warm up with Dynamic Stretching and warm down with Static Stretching and foam rolling, take Epsom salt baths.

There are also ways you can tell if it's a good soreness or bad. Say your biceps are sore from an arm workout the day before. If your bicep is sore to the touch I would consider that a good soreness. If you are feeling soreness in the tendons that attach to the bicep muscle, then it would be a good idea to get out of the gym and give it a rest! That would be something I would not want to work through and can be more harmful than good!

Be smart and listen to your body. Recovery and Overtraining kind of go hand in hand. There are signs that your body gives you to tell you that you need to rest. Unless you are a competitive athlete, you must develop the skill of listening to your body and do exactly what it says.

Here are some of the signs that tell you that you are overtraining:

- Insomnia
- Prolonged muscle soreness
- Increased Resting Metabolic Heart Rate
- Loss of appetite
- Increased incidence of injuries
- Irritability
- Depression
- Loss of motivation

If you are experiencing any of these symptoms for a period of time, take off a few days and see what happens. I'll bet you will come back stronger than ever.

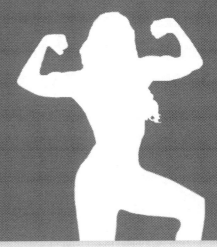

CHAPTER 8

LIFE AFTER COMPETITIVE BODYBUILDING

In 2003, I donated my kidney to my Aunt Carol Presley, a precious soul.

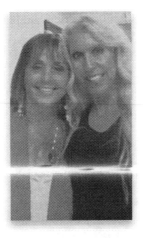

She passed away in June 2017. That operation had me down for a long time and I was very anxious to get back to my fitness regimen. When the surgery was performed they discovered a hernia which I had no idea I had. Recovery was difficult but I made it through just fine without any complications. Fitness had become a lifestyle for me. Remember, I'm infected. I wanted so badly to make it my sole income but it just wasn't happening. Not then anyway.

In 2004 I married Mike Crall. I was working in retail management at the time and lived in Hope, Arkansas. I met Mike in 2002 on a dating site. I didn't put my picture on the site simply because I didn't want to be thrown into the meat market, so to speak. I was looking for someone sincere, clean non bar hopper and non smoker. I found his bio with his picture so I "winked" at him and he "winked" back. We started conversing online and our conversations were very basic. We talked about what we did that day, our favorite movies and music and things like that. He never asked me for my phone number but offered his. I never called. After a few weeks I finally sent him a picture. We continued to talk online then I discovered I had overlooked an important characteristic. He was a smoker. I thought to myself, OH NO! How did I miss this? I told him that I was sorry but I didn't know he smoked. That's going to be a problem, I said. We talked about it and came to an agreement that he would never smoke in my presence. Deal. We continued to communicate. Two months later he asked me on a date. There was a four hour distance between us but he drove four hours to meet me for dinner at Texas Roadhouse in Texarkana, Tx. After dinner he drove back home. The rest is history! I love you Mike Crall. Thank you for picking me to be your wife.

In 2008, I started working full time for a Fitness Center in Hurst, Texas as a personal trainer. I drove 30-45 minutes one-way to work every day. This work was fun and I gained a lot of experience and got re-certified as a personal trainer. I worked a 40-hour week and literally had no real time to train my self. When I did squeeze in a workout I was too exhausted to really give it what I needed and wanted and I had put on a few pounds. I was working in Fitness. It's where I wanted to be right? Right. I just needed to find that balance between me and work.

Having my own fitness studio had been a long time goal of mine. I started doing my homework by asking questions and seeking counsel. I had been told that it would take at least $70,000 to open up the type of fitness facility that I wanted. The person who said this to me obviously didn't know me. I just knew I could do it and make it profitable enough. I wanted it and was determined to make it happen. I just didn't have $70k to start and did not want a loan!

Boot Camps

In 2009, I began teaching boot camps in the park on my off days and business was booming. I operated out of a little red wagon and had a battle rope, cones and weights.

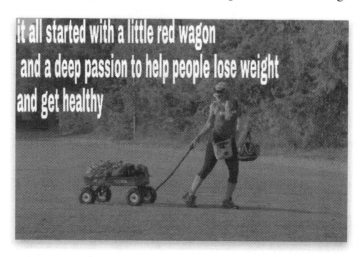

(Compliments of Lynn Murdock of Image Maker Pix Photography)

It was proving profitable, but it didn't stay that way. You see, I learned fast that 85% of people who start an exercise program end up falling out for a variety of reasons. That's just the stats people. It's fitness and that's just the way it is. I started working out in 1981 and I have been very consistent but few people obtain this type of crazy motivation and it takes crazy motivation to make it happen and stay motivated.

I was FEARLESS in the pursuit of what set my soul on fire. FITNESS! I made the boot camps work around my hours at my other job until they closed the doors at the gym. Another set back. I had to find another income because I knew how fitness worked and knew that I had to learn a few more things before I took my next big move.

Another full time job came in retail management and I was able to continue my boot camps but had to cut way back due to my hours at my new job. I didn't want to wake up in the mornings to go to work. I fell into a pattern. All I did was come home and complain about my "job." But I didn't give up. I had a goal and knew I had to keep working towards that. I still had this crazy motivation even when I was miserable. I always had 100% total support from my husband in anything I wanted to do and his continuing patience of a monk and support had helped me grow into who I am today.

The Birth Of Boot Camp Academy 101 Fitness Studio

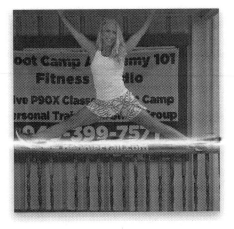

I continued in my mission and in 2011, I decided to take the leap of faith. I found a vacant hole in the wall and took a peak inside. It was a mess but I saw potential and I had to put my creative mind to work. I called the owner and she met me there and after speaking with her I decided that it would not work. There was too much money involved and too much work to do to get this place ready. I continued to look. Two months later she called and asked if I had thought anymore about it. I decided to look at it one more time. I called my honey and he met me over there and we signed a lease.

October 2011, I opened the doors to "Boot Camp Academy 101 Fitness Studio." Now, here is the funny part. I opened my studio with a few dumbbells, a cheap weight bench, a couple of

Medicine balls and some bands. I gradually increased my inventory over time. It cracked me up when the Chamber of Commerce came out to cut the ribbon. They were shocked to see so little equipment in there. Someone asked, where are all the machines? I told them that I AM the machine. We laughed and I cut the ribbon.

I learned quickly that I didn't need a bunch of high dollar equipment that shines like the top of the Chrysler building and I didn't want to do what the average fitness owner did either. I didn't want to follow the rules of running my own business. For example, I didn't like the idea of auto deduction for payment. That's what set me apart from the other fitness places in town. I knew it was a risk but I took it anyway. Someone made the comment that if I didn't set my members up on auto deduct, I wouldn't last more than 2 years. I was completely confident that my way made sense. I offered what was rare to find in other businesses. A heart and soul. A smile and big hello when they walked in the door. Something to make them feel welcome and warm.

These women came to associate with others and connect with like-minded people and to get/ stay healthy and to make friends. Women needed that connection and BCA101 offered that. It became increasingly difficult keeping up with everyone on social media but I did it. It was the only way I could find out what they were going through in life. Was it a death, a child's birthday, honeymoon, wedding, vacation, etc... I wanted to acknowledge everyone. I never had a lot of money, but I always had a passion and a heart that truly cares about people.

At first I offered classes and boot camps. I was teaching seventeen classes a week and there was literally no time for anything else but I was so happy being where I was. Eventually, I canceled the lowest attendant classes and started adding Personal Training and Small Group. Whenever I became discouraged I would look back and picture everything I went through to get there. I knew up front and without a doubt that it would be hard work but I was ready. I loved it and I was literally celebrating.

DID YOU KNOW: If you give someone a smile nine times out ten you will get one back. So smile at someone today! Make their day. You may be the only one who does.

Burn Out

Someone asked me if I ever get tired? My response, you bet I do. I take a 5-10 minute power nap on most days. I eat for energy and get plenty of rest, but yes I do get tired. Their next question was, don't you get burnt out? I said, no. Tired yes, burnt out, no. Well, it came later but I set myself up for that without knowing it. I remember in one National Academy of Sports Medicine Personal Training workshop I attended that if you do everything in your business yourself, you are setting yourself up for burn out. I thought, nah, not me. I was wrong. I was everything - the Trainer, the bookkeeper, the cleaning lady, the marketer, the psychologist, the advertiser, the program designer, social media advertiser, the nutrition advisor. Everything. I eventually hired help but if you've ever had a business before you will understand this phrase: Good people are hard to find.

Burn out for me came five years later. It became increasingly difficult for me to maintain any sort of personal fitness regimen myself. I was giving everything I had to everyone else.

I closed the doors of Boot Camp Academy 101 in October 2016 and a load was dropped from my shoulders. I started working out again at a local fitness facility and finally invested back into me.

Boot Camp Academy 101 Fitness Studio was an extremely successful business. In 2015 Boot Camp Academy 101 Fitness Studio was voted #1 as the best fitness facility in Decatur, Texas.

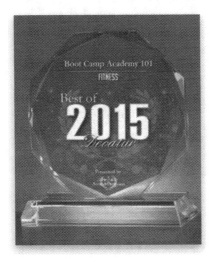

BCA101 JOURNEY:

In 2014, Netflix did a documentary "FEARLESS" featuring me as the personal trainer for 3 time PBR World Champion Bull Rider, Silvano Alves.

See a clip of Silvano's training program on my youtube channel.

In 2015 I appeared in an episode on RDF TV offering exercise tips to a world renowned barrel racer to keep her core tight and riding strong.

In 2015 I tried out for and trained for American Ninja Warrior. Even though they never put me on the show I was asked to test some of the new obstacles in Houston, Texas and St. Louis, Missouri. An adventure I will never forget! My momma went with me to St. Louis to watch!

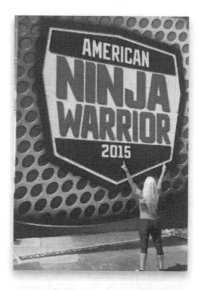

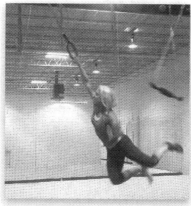

My training for this obstacle course was at Obstacle Warriors in Dallas, Texas, owners Samantha and Robert Reid. They offer pretty much everything a competitor would need in terms of obstacle training and a lot of kid activities. Monkey bars were always my favorite.

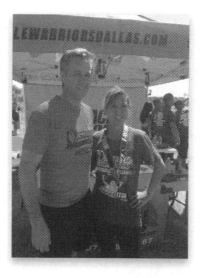

LiveIt Magazine featured me in their January/February 2016 issue on health and fitness.

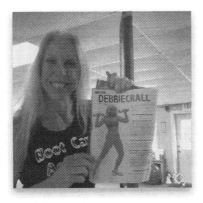

Boot Camp Academy 101 Fitness Studio brought me a ton of experience and a ton of good memories. I met a lot of wonderful people.

CHAPTER 9

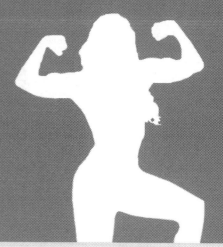

FEMALE BODYBUILDING SUPPORTED

I ran an advertisement in a local newspaper one time advertising my boot camps. I received an offensive text message on my cell phone from an unknown person. They asked me if that was a man in the ad. I don't answer stupid questions but it still disturbs me that ignorance of this magnitude still permeates the population. I could see this person lacked a tremendous amount of knowledge about weight training.

I'll have to admit I am a little larger, somewhat stronger and a lot more sculpted than the average woman. I had a plan thirty-five plus years ago to redesign my pear shape into a more symmetrical body. I did that through BODYBUILDING. As a bodybuilder, you no doubt place a premium on you appearance. That's the name of the game. But why is there so misconception on this subject?

The answer may be due to competitive bodybuilders themselves, both men and women. They are just getting bigger and bigger, disregarding symmetry all together. Many gave up pursuing extreme bodybuilding and the International Federation of Bodybuilding took notice and shifted the aesthetics back to the classic bodybuilding days of thirty years ago where women and men have a more flattering look of a nice streamline and perfect muscular proportions. I believe people view these muscled up women and men on the front of muscle magazines and automatically judge them.

This extreme type of modern bodybuilding seems more about presentation and less about fitness. This is primarily expressed by newcomers to the sport. Granted, more and more women are turning to bodybuilding as a quick way to shape up, but there are still a few who are afraid of the word. Some fear that BODYBUILDING means bulking up like the power lifter.

A power lifter's goal is to become stronger. A bodybuilder's goal is to enhance her appearance to create a shapely streamline. If you want to compete and show off your hard work, so be it.

There is also a process you go through regarding carbohydrates to prep for a show and this is called Peaking. Once you reach your peak, it better be on judgment day because it only lasts 24 hours. Then you begin to soften up a bit. This is all a part of competing. Along with BODYBUILDING training you will become stronger and more flexible. You will also reduce your body fat and obtain better cardiovascular fitness.

Do all the aerobics you want, run ten miles a day if you wish, but nothing is going to reshape and tighten your body like bodybuilding can. So you may ask, is bodybuilding for me? All I can say is, put on that bikini, stand in front of a full-length mirror and look at you from all angles. Do you like what you see? If not, bodybuilding is for you!

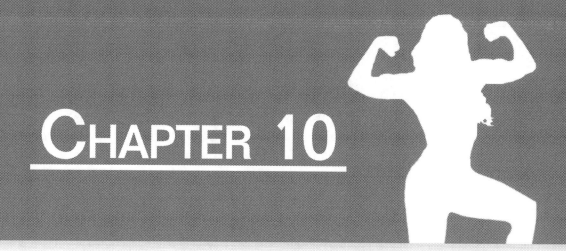

CHAPTER 10

NUTRITION FOR ATHLETES

There are literally tons of supplements on the market today.

During my competitive years I took amino acids before and after my workouts, and still do, to help with recovery and to limit muscle breakdown. I was really big on taking vitamins B-Complex and C during competition. Today I include a joint supplement and calcium.

My daily nutrition plan includes well-balanced proportions of protein/carbs/fats and I eat for energy. After logging and making detailed notes for two years, I now know how a certain food will make me feel and look. Unless you are a professional athlete in training you know that it takes a certain amount of nutrients to get through those tough training sessions. I could not eat like I did back during my competitive days and be as lean as I am now simply because I'm not using those extra calories posing and training twice a day. A lot of calories are burned during preparation.

Here is an example of a typical day I adhered to during my competitive days:

8-10 weeks out from a show (4,000 calories a day)

- 5am oatmeal/ 6 egg whites/2 pieces toast
- Train 6a-7a
- 7:30 2 chicken breast/veggies
- 9:30 6 egg white omelette with veggies
- 10:30-11:30 Posing/tanning
- 11:30am oatmeal/broccoli/2 slices toast
- 1:30 tuna sandwich/salad
- 3:30: homemade Protein Shake

- 5:30-6:30 train
- 8pm 6 Egg white omelette with veggies
- 9pm bedtime

This worked really well for me. Test your body and see what works for you. Above all, know your metabolism. Nowadays, there are some competitors that do what they call water pull a couple of days before a show which I think is totally nuts. No water?? But hey, if it works for you and you are not dead, go for it. I no longer log my food but know depending on my daily activity what I need to eat to maintain not only my body weight but my energy level.

If you are preparing for a competition, on judgment day, you better be on because the peak only lasts about 24 hours. When you peak you look tight and full on stage. After about 24 hours, you begin to soften up a bit and start losing your pump, which is what happened to me at the show in Dallas in 2016. I was at my best 2 weeks before that show. I would like to point out that it's during these times where people get a big misconception on bodybuilding. They see these huge muscles and veins but what they don't know is we don't walk around like this all the time. We would all be dead! But, the word bodybuilding does get a bad wrap especially from the women. Some actually fear of becoming too bulky and everyones opinion on "bulky" is different. People who are new to the sport of bodybuilding primarily express this fear.

I had a plan 35 plus years ago to redesign my pear shape into a more symmetrical body. I corrected that through BODYBUILDING and proper nutrition, not drugs. Bodybuilding will change your shape dramatically and that was what I set out to do.

Nutrition and its Role in Fitness

I get bombarded with questions about what to eat before a workout, what to eat after a workout, what can I eat as a snack, should I take supplements, etc. These are all million dollar questions and I honestly believe that once you understand that everyone is different you will be on a mission to find what works for you. What works for others may not work for you.

I can tell you that I have found what works for me after logging my food for two years straight. I know exactly what a food will have me feeling like and looking like. I know what foods to avoid and what foods I can have on occasion.

I know a few people who thrive on their own special diets, whether it's low carbohydrate, high carbohydrate, high protein, vegan etc. and there are a lot of people who don't. This can be confusing when searching the Internet for the perfect diet. You may find a website that says to eat carbohydrates before a workout and another one say eat protein before a workout. It can be confusing but it doesn't have to be. Again, your body is a science, so do your homework. If you have tried a diet that didn't work for you, try something else. Try eating more vegetables. Try keeping a log along with detailed notes after your meal. Educate yourself as much as you possibly can and read everything regarding nutrition and fitness that you can get your hands on.

More importantly, make this long term vs short term results! If you're reading this book that means you are educating yourself. Congratulations, you are one step closer. Continue to research and sooner or later you will find out what works for you. This is what is takes. When you find what is working, be consistent. I can't stress this enough.

Consistency takes the cake. You may not be the type to log your food but I strongly recommend it. It's your homework. It's your science project and it's like a science test. Is it easy? No. But neither was that science test you took in school. It's the only way you can see what's working and what's not and it will be well worth your while. Coffee is always on the menu for me and I do better working out on empty but not starving. Some people can have a big breakfast and hit the gym with no problem. I'd get sick if I did this but, again, that's me. Find out what works for you.

I used the Nutrition Almanac by John D. Kirschmann, Director, with Lavon J. Dunne as I was learning, logging and making detailed notes on how I felt after eating. I still refer to this on occasion and highly recommend this book if you want to know your body inside and out. More on nutrition books in Chapter 14.

My Sweet Tooth

My weakness is donuts and every 3-4 weeks I'll have one or two donuts. Cream filled maple bars and glazed donuts are my favorite. It's crazy funny how your clients see you around town and you are busted eating a donut. I received a text once after driving through Braum's Ice Cream one day getting a frozen strawberry mix. The text said what are you eating at Braum's that is so healthy? I replied, a Strawberry Mix, don't judge me. Often times I feel like I need to hide so people don't think I do this all the time. Understand there's a fine line in doing this once every 2-3 weeks and eating like this every day. Everything in moderation.

Society has conditioned our taste buds to crave fatty, salty, sugary foods. You can practically swing your purse walking through town and hit a fast food restaurant. It is becoming crazy. So if you are a fast food eater, what you must do is de-condition your taste buds. Plan your meals and do all the prepping at home so you'll know what you are getting. It'll take a little discipline but you can do it. Here are some tips for you to put into practice…

- Have regular meals. In addition to keeping your metabolism high, eating small meals helps keep calorie intake low. Don't starve yourself
- Try to Eat in a calm and relaxed atmosphere if you can control it. Never eat angry. It alters your digestion.
- Take time and chew your food

- Put a limit on your shopping and make your food choices wisely. Bring home only foods that will help you contribute to a healthy diet. Ok, now listen, I'm not saying never
- have a cookie, or piece of cake or ice cream. I'm saying make at least 90% of your
- calories clean, wholesome nutrient filled foods
- Shop online for recipes and get creative. I personally like allrecipes.com.
- Learn how to read labels in the store and what to look for. More on label reading later.
- Learn to cook. Use spices for flavor versus the salt shaker.
- Make cooking easy and FUN!
- Prep your meals ahead of time and plan your days. Be prepared.
- Mealtime is actually the best part of my day. It's easy for me simply because I plan.
- If you go to a party, plan it to where its that 10% day…90% healthy and 10% partyfood. Don't go overboard though. Just because it's your 10% doesn't mean it's a license to pig out. Be wise about it and remember it's all about conditioning your taste buds.
- Enjoy your favorite meal every once in awhile for Pete's sake! Just portion it out and don't stuff yourself.
- Drink plenty of water.

If you live on the road all you can do is plan and make better choices.

CHAPTER 11

SODIUM AND FOOD LABELING

Check with your doctor on this as well as anything having to do with nutrition.

According to National Academy of Sports Medicine, a healthy individual, salt/sodium should range from 1800 to 2400 mg per day. Salt saps calcium from the bones, weakening them over time. For every 2,300 milligrams of sodium you take in, you lose about 40 milligrams of calcium, so some dieticians claim. One study compared postmenopausal women who ate a high-salt diet with those who didn't, and the ones who ate a lot of salt lost more bone minerals.

Our American diet is salt-heavy sugar-ladened and ridiculous. Most people ingest triple the 2,400 milligrams of sodium we should get in one day and probably don't even know it simply because they don't know how to read labels at the grocery store. How much sodium are you eating? Do you know? Now, I'm not asking you if you add salt to your food. I'm asking you if you know how much sodium you are eating on a daily basis. Put that pen to paper and watch it get real. Yes, we all need some sodium for good health. However, the average American diet contains about three times more sodium than is healthy, which leads to high blood pressure and other health issues.

What to do: The quickest, most efficient way to cut back on sodium is to avoid processed foods and fast food. Key foods to avoid include processed and deli meats, frozen meals, canned soup and vegetables, pizza, fast food. Restaurant foods are the culprits for the high levels of sodium in today's diets. Just because it says heart healthy doesn't mean it is. Do your homework and ask for nutritional Information on it. Don't be shy. Ask!

Food Labeling

This isn't rocket science and requires no degree. Once you become aware of reading labels it will become easier for you to make better choices. Learn to look beyond the buzzwords and fancy claims on the front of the eye catching box. Learn how to read between the lines of the marketing spin. I am forever comparing products with catchy labels. Most of it is the eye-catching label that makes me pick it up and flip it over to read the label. People shop at the grocery store looking for the latest buzzword. For example, fat free, no sugar added, no salt added, low sodium, all natural, made with real fruit, zero trans fat, heart healthy, organic, low carb, etc…

Manufacturers will try to lure you into buying their product. They can't lie to you about the nutrition and ingredients of their products, but they can easily mislead you into thinking something is healthier than it really is. Know the difference. It's a law that food labels must tell the truth. However, manufactures can pick and choose which facts to highlight and spin so they catch your attention. How many people actually flip it over and read the label? Do research on it. Study. Remember, your body is a science project and you are putting things to the test and learning.

Trips out of town are used as an excuse constantly. I understand sometimes things get in the way that deters you from your workouts and eating healthy. If you don't have time, the least you can do is make better choices to de-condition those tastebuds. I used to eat Cheeseburgers, boxed cereals, canned vegetables and fruit and drink Dr Pepper like crazy. The more I became aware of my bad habits, I slowly began to make some changes by cutting back on some things. Instead of five Dr Peppers a day, I did four. Then three. Then eventually cutting them out 100%. It's all about the taste buds and your desire to change. Don't make change too complicated. Just begin.

How I keep it together on a tight schedule: I schedule any appointments around meals and workouts, if I can help it. Waiting until the last minute will have you grabbing for anything. So planning is crucial if you want serious results.

When I go on road trips, I don't have the luxury of prepping my own meals but I do have the ability to make better choices. For example, I want salt. I'm looking at Pringles but Bugles look pleasing too. I'm reading the labels and pick the best choice. Which one would you pick? There is your first assignment.

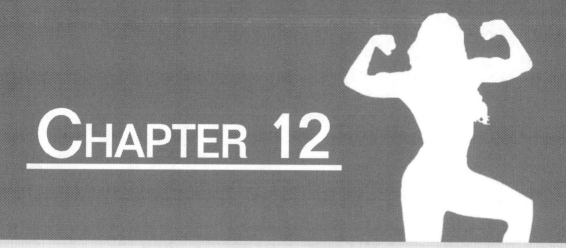

CHAPTER 12

PROTEIN & AMINO ACIDS

Amino Acids do several things.

1. Speeds up muscle repair.
2. Promotes Muscle Growth.
3. Limits Muscle Breakdown.

Recommended Protein Intake

Ask your doctor first.

National Academy of Sports Medicine recommends the following:

AVERAGE PERSON 0.8 grams per kg body weight for the average person and it is also recommended that 15-25% of your daily calories should come from protein.

ENDURANCE ATHLETES : Protein

1.2 - 1.4 grams per kg body weight

STRENGTH ATHLETES: Protein

1.6 - 1.7 grams per kg body weight.

Carbohydrates

Recommended Intake of Carbohydrates

Be sure and ask your doctor when embarking on a no carbohydrate diet. According to National Academy of Sports Medicine it is recommended that the average body needs 45% - 65% of their total calories from carbohydrates, primarily as complex carbohydrates. Keep in mind this is based on your activities. Carbohydrates are a much needed nutrient and should fluctuate depending on your daily activities.

Inactive individuals only need around 3 grams per kg body weight per day.

Example:

60 x 3 = 180 grams per day.

Active individuals (those who exercise 45 minutes - 1 hour) need 4-5 grams per kg body weight per day.

Example:

60 x 5 = 300 grams per day

Athletes who training with high intensely may need as much as 8-12 grams per kg body weight.

Example:

60kg x 12 = 720 grams per day.

I personally cycle my carbohydrates. Meaning I'm at the upper end (12 grams per kg bodyweight) if I'm planning on an intense workout. On my active rest days, it is the lower end of the scale. I'm blessed with a speedy metabolism. Thanks, mom and dad.

The recommendations provide a place to begin, but you must find what works for you since everyone is different.

COMPLEX CARBOHYDRATE EXAMPLES:

Grains, wheat, rice, corn, oats, potatoes, pasta, peas.

Soluble Fiber: Nuts, apples, blueberries, oatmeal, beans

Insoluble Fiber: Bran, Brown rice, fruit skins

CARBOHYDRATES ARE IMPORTANT FUEL DURING A WORKOUT.

Again, ask your doctor.

Simple carbohydrates are found naturally in foods such as fruits, milk, and milk products. They are also found in processed and refined sugars such as candy, table sugar, syrups, and soft drinks, breads and cereal.

Fat And It's Functions

Fat gives you energy too, just like carbohydrates. They store your energy and protect and insulate your vital organs. There is good fat and bad fat.

National Academy of Sports Medicine recommend you follow these guidelines:

- Eat these foods frequently: Non-starchy veggies, raw leafy green veggies, solid green veggies.
- Use portion control on these: Starchy vegetables, whole grains, raw nuts and seeds, fish, fat free dairy, poultry, eggs
- Eat these very sparingly: Red meat, full-fat dairy, cheese, refined grains, crackers, chips, white pasta, oils, etc,
- refined sweets like, baked goodies, candy and soda.

I started making really good gains when I finally learned how to eat!

CHAPTER 13

GIMMICKS AND FADS

This is the most misinformed and 'fueled by myths society' that I have ever encountered.

Everything seems to revolve around the latest trend. The sad thing is people are falling for the latest trend and often surrendering their health and fitness. False information and the latest trends will continue to thrive in the minds of people because the companies that are pushing these gimmicks are making money. A LOT of money! It is a six billion dollar industry and they know and understand the weakness of the obese. People desire a rapid way to better health. These people fall for anything hook line and sinker and steadily jumping for those catchy phrases.

- Dramatic weight loss (30 pounds in 30 days)
- One easy permanent solution
- Just take this pill or use this patch, cream… for Amazing Results
- Buy this food or supplement
- The miracle diet

I personally do not trust anything that does not encourage permanent lifestyle changes and I have trust issues with anything that is highly advertised. Be smart and do your homework and just because everyone else is doing this doesn't mean it will work for you. It may work in the beginning but if you can't keep it off, something is wrong. Get yourself an app that you can track your calories with and don't eat more than that! Period. No better way to reach your goal than to teach yourself about your own body and how to nourish it. Know where you are going or you will end up somewhere else.

I have read many diet/nutrition books as mentioned earlier. I still read nutrition and fitness magazines. Things change and new science information are discovered. I have tried a variety of different supplement lines. I took the journey down the path of amino acids capsules, amino acid drinks, energy drinks, etc. until I realized there is no shortcut to anyplace worth going. Just learn how to eat and exercise. No big secret here. No magic pill that is going to teach you how to eat. You must do this yourself. Your body is your science project so do your homework and get your macronutrients in order. If you are using a supplement line and it's working for you, obviously this does not apply to you.

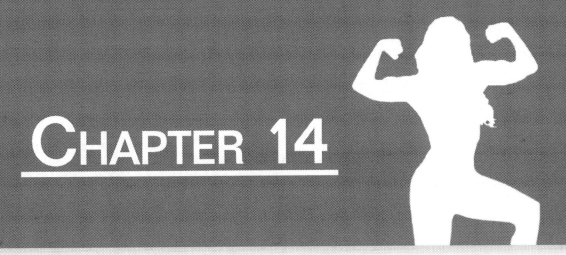

NUTRITION BOOKS

The Nutrition Almanac

Nutrition Search Inc., John D. Kirschmann, Director, with Lavon J. Dunne. This book covers in detail nutrition and health, sources of calories, nutrients and how they function together. The book also contains expanded, easy - to - read food composition chart, ailments, stressful conditions, nutrition and Herbs. I literally lived out of this book when I started training for competitions. I learned a tremendous amount from Doug and Jeannie as well.

Eat Right For Your Type

Dr. Peter J. D'Adamo with Catherine Whitney. The Blood Type Diet is a complete blood type encyclopedia. It teaches you how to treat everything from asthma to thrombosis, allergies to sore throats and even cancer. You can treat over three hundred conditions utilizing the right remedy for your blood type.

Fit For Life

Harvey and Marilyn Diamond with a forward by Edward Taub, M.D. This is another book that is a welcomed addition to my library. This book discusses your natural body cycles, Appropriation Cycle, Assimilation and Elimination Cycle and the pitfalls of combining macro-nutrients. This book is all about food combining.

Nutrition For Dummies 3Rd Addition

Carol Ann Rinser, Author of <u>Controlling Cholesterol For Dummies</u>. This one is about making wise food choices and teaches you how to maintain a healthy lifestyle.

None of these books requires you to take this pill, or apply this patch, or drink this or that. These are hard-core nutritional facts that teach you how to eat. Learn your body needs.

CHAPTER 15

SPECIAL POPULATIONS AND WHERE TO BEGIN

Most exercise guidelines are designed specifically for healthy individuals between 18 and 65 years of age. Resistance training among older adults can be very rewarding, highly beneficial and should be recommended as per your doctor. Modifications are definitely in order for the healthy, senior citizen. For example, a push up for a healthy 20-30 year old would obviously look entirely different for a relatively healthy senior citizen. A skilled trainer can provide anyone with a good overall conditioning and flexibility fitness plan. I believe everyone should strive for this no matter what your age. It is never too late.

Where to Begin an Exercise Progam.

Let me first mention one very important component of physical fitness. The psoas, pronounced: 'So As'. The Psoas is the epitome of the CORE. The abdominal muscles are included but they are out on the superficial layer of the body. So when you look at the core, you are looking at the spine and the muscles closest to it, which includes the PSOAS. It also sits on our center of gravity. This is the key to PSOAS in terms of movement. Basic function of the muscle is walking - putting one foot in front of the other. A lot of what we do from day to day involve throwing our center of gravity around. Every move you make, every step you take, every bend, twist, reach involves your center of gravity and focus is key.

Stabilization /Phase 1

To start off, your goal should be to increase muscle endurance and this requires some patience. You may not think you are doing anything because the muscles you are working on are not superficial, like biceps and quadriceps! These are deep muscles and joints that must be strong enough so you can take it to the next level. Some people, particularly senior citizens stay in this phase and it is totally ok! The object of the game is to strengthen the Core and Core Movement System.

Three days a week is all you need for the first 4-6 weeks if you are just starting out. Then increase your progress to 4-5 days a week, if you choose to. This highly depends on what your fitness goals are and your limitations. Below are some suggestions for strengthening and progressions.

ISO AB ON STABILITY BALL (hold: 30) If you can master this for 30 seconds with no issues you are then ready to challenge yourself.

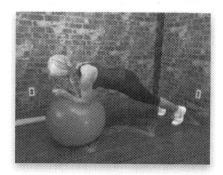

1 LEG PRONE HIP EXT (10 repetitions on each side)

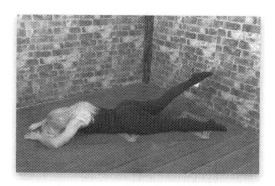

COBRA (10 -12 reps) (10 repetitions on each side)

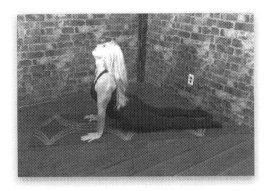

SIDE PLANK (10 reps)

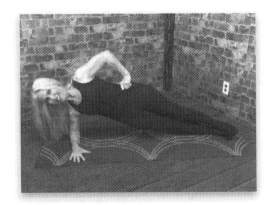

- PROGRESS GRADUALLY BY ADDING ONE OF THE FOLLOWING AFTER 3-4 WEEKS
- SEATED TWIST

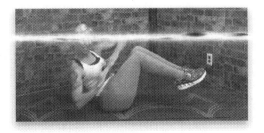

- STABILITY BALL CRUNCH

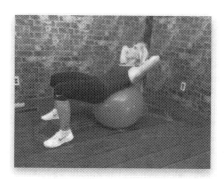

Functional training is what happens in the real world. It's all based on our body mechanics and how we move throughout the day. We lift things up. We set things down. We bend over and pick things up. We reach. We twist. We turn. We walk. We sit and stand. Functional exercises are very beneficial for everyone, no matter your age or what type of training you do, this should be included at least once to twice a week. Here are some excellent functional exercises to strengthen your joints and keep them strong.

1-3 sets/ 10 repetitions:

1 LEG BICEP CURL

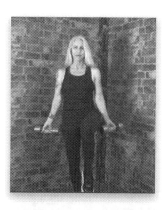

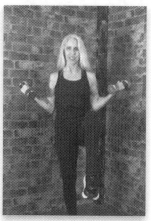

1 LEG OVERHEAD PRESS

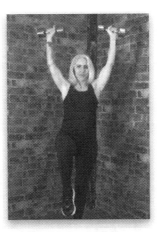

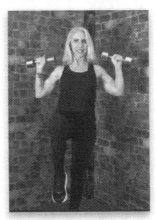

Strength Endurance /Phase 2

Perhaps you want to consider adding to your workout, jumping rope or marching in place for 1 minute, fast walking or jogging for 10-20 minutes, jogging outside or on the treadmill or stair master.

My cardio choice is a bit different than the average. I choose to do a non-stop weight training session for my cardio. Treadmills and Ellipticals bore me! In weight training, you continue to burn more calories after you stop training. If you were to hit the pavement running, you pretty much stop burning calories when you stop the activity. Try doing a little weight training and then head out for a run or fast walk. If you stick to what you enjoy, your chances of staying consistent will be better. If you prefer the treadmill, stair master, elliptical cardio equipment, go for that.

The endurance phase will require higher repetitions and lower loads, 2-4 sets in a giant set. I love doing giant sets. I group four exercises together and do them back-to-back, rest and repeat. Here is a good one for legs:

4 giant sets/ 25 reps without breaking my reps up. In other words, 25 non-stop squats, dead lifts, lunges and single leg dead lifts.

Do these back to back, rest and repeat for four total round making it four giant sets. You can choose any body part you want to do with giant sets, I just love hitting the legs like this and you probably will as well.

Hypertrophy/ Phase 3

3-5 sets per exercise

6-12 reps.

This has got to be my favorite way to train. Even though I love it so much, doesn't mean I train in this phase all the time. As previously mentioned, I mix it up a lot. Anyway, Hypertrophy means, enlargement of muscles. The workload is approximately 85% intensity for 3-5 sets. Remember, Phase 1 and 2 are used to prepare your muscles and joints for this type of workout load. Also, nutrition plays a huge roll in building significant muscle size. More on repetitions and sets in Chapter 17.

Gaining Muscle

If your goal is to gain muscle size, pick a weight that will challenge you - a weight you can do 6-12 reps with, in good form, making sure your last few reps are an all out effort. Train intensely and be consistent.

Afraid of Becoming Too Big and Toning

Actually, this concept is the same thing just with a different understanding. What do you think your doing when you lift a weight up and use it? You are building muscle. If you reach a point where you are scared to lift a heavy weight for fear of becoming bulky, I am here to tell you this does not happen overnight. Any experienced bodybuilder will tell you the same thing. Progressions come very slowly so patience is key. The beautiful thing about bodybuilding is you can scale back when you reach your goal and start maintaining.

Nutrition will play a big role too. It took me literally years to reach a point where I wanted to start maintaining. It is how I train today. Yes, I go heavy and train hard but my diet does not include gaining any significant amount of muscle size. In addition, as I age, I do not want to lose those type 2 muscle fibers. I train with low reps at times for power to stress the type 2 muscle fibers.

CHAPTER 16

OBESITY/ LIPOSUCTION AND COSMETIC SURGERY

I have never had cosmetic surgery of any kind or liposuction nor do I see it as an option in my future. I am the most blessed egg my momma has ever hatched and was born with good genetics. Those not so fortunate can look at a candy bar and gain weight while others can eat five or six candy bars and not gain an ounce. I can't help that, but you can do the best you can with what you have. More importantly, do not use that as your excuse.

There are ways to rev up the metabolism to burn fat and it is really quite simple. Turn off the TV, move more and eat clean. If you want to get a jump-start on your journey and your doctor advises it, I'm all for cosmetic surgery if your health is at risk and you are morbidly obese or look just want a jump-start on your fitness journey. I support this 100%. However, I don't support it as a means of being lazy and not doing what you are required to do after the surgery. I know several people that have gone through Lap Ban two times simply because they refuse to exercise and eat right. They had the surgery, lost a bunch of weight and gained it right back and more because they are - in a word - lazy. Perhaps, it is simply education; they just don't know how to eat. Get the surgery if you are called to do that, feel confident in your skin and when you recover, get to work.

Obesity

Obesity is on the rise and it is now considered a "Chronic Disease." It has become a serious health problem! Helping an individual lose weight is a taunting task for most personal trainers! We have control over what goes on in the workouts. We can advise them on what to do outside the sessions. But, ultimately they are responsible! All I can do is teach them to make better choices.

We are having an obesity explosion. Our plates are loaded! And, all the fast food, sweet drinks, high calorie desserts has not only filled us up, but OUT! Statistics indicate that 1 in every 3 children and adults are obese or overweight.

FIT TIPS: Use smaller plates. Stop eating when you are full. Drink water before your meal. Cut way back on fast food. Learn to read labels and make better choices at the grocery store and practice portion control.

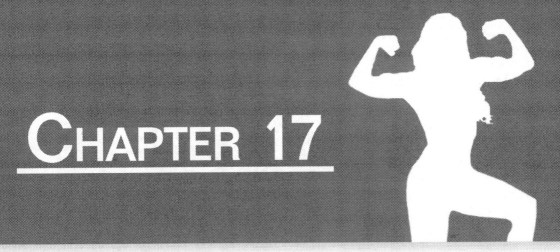

CHAPTER 17

REPETITION AND SETS

A Repetition is how many times you perform the exercise without stopping.

A Set is how many rounds you complete.

EXAMPLE:

3 sets of 10 repetitions would look like this:

First set: 10 pushups without stopping.

Second set: Rest and repeat 10 repetitions without stopping

Third set: Rest and repeat 10 repetitions without stopping.

You've just completed 3 sets of 10 repetitions on push-ups.

Training Volume will vary widely depending on what you want to accomplish in your fitness program and if you are training for a specific athletic event. My training volume changes all the time depending on my energy level. One workout may consist of chest, shoulders and triceps. I may do 12 sets for 6-12 reps for each muscle group: chest, shoulders and triceps and it might look something like this:

PICK YOUR OWN WEIGHT. The weight you select must be challenging enough to create a neuromuscular response.

Push Ups 3-4 sets of 6-12 repetitions

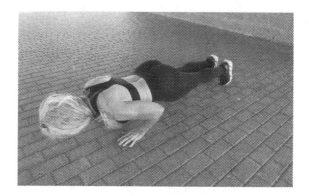

Overhead Press 3-4 sets of 6-12- repetitions

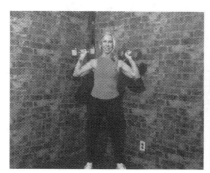 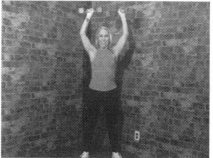

Side Laterals 3-4 sets of 6-12 repetitions

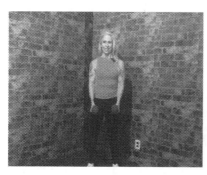 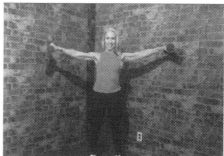

Bent Over Row 3-4 sets of 6-12 repetitions

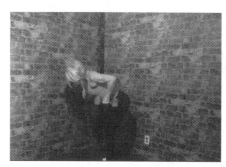 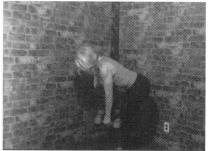

Front Raises 3-4 sets of 6-12 repetitions

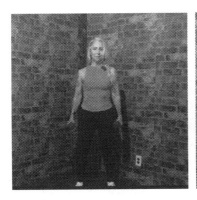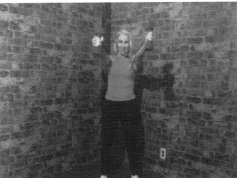

Dips 3-4 sets of 6-12 repetitions

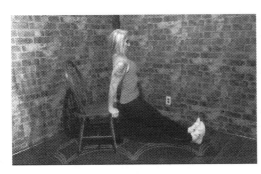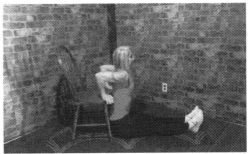

Kickbacks 3-4 sets of 6-12 repetitions

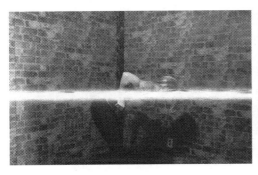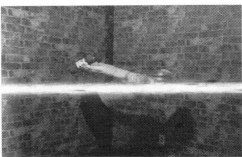

Some days I may do high reps, some days Tabata style and some days Breakdowns, Pyramid training and other days I go super light and perform high reps. Nothing is ever carved in stone.

I also change up my training by doing a superset or I have a little circuit going on and may decide to vary my workouts Cross fit style. Every one of my workouts is different and varies constantly. This is what I recommend you do if you want body composition results, unless you are training for a specific sport.

Training Volume and Rest Periods

Always remember that when your training volume decreases, your load volume increases. Here is a great example of what I'm talking about:

If you train 85 to 90% of your 1 Rep Max, I consider that a very intense workout. The next time you are not real energized so you work at say 65-70% of your 1 Rep Max. Chances are you are using super light weights at 70% meaning you are recovering a lot faster than the day you worked at 85-95% with super heavy weights simply because it is a lot less taxing on the nervous system verses when you train heavy. When I'm going heavy, which is what I do most of the time, my rest period will be anywhere from 1-2 minutes. Just enough to recover my ATP cellular energy at least 80% and my workout is done in 35-45 minutes. If you are consistently spending anymore than an hour to an hour and a half in the gym and if you are not a pro athlete training for an event, you need to probably re-evaluate your workout program.

Consistency

Consistency takes the cake. There are rewards from consistency you will not find anywhere else. I understand things come up in life to keep you from staying on track. It certainly has happened to me, but overall your training and nutrition should be as consistent as you can possibly make it. Pick a time and day that works for you and stick with it. Plan your meals. Schedule your doctor's appointments around your workouts if you can help it. Working out consistently for three days and taking off two weeks will not get you any significant results. If you want to maintain, you need at least three days a week of consistent training. Schedule more time if you want serious results. Work into it slowly. Make it a habit like brushing your teeth.

CHAPTER 18

THE DESK JOB AND MUSCLE IMBALANCES

Does your typical day look like this?

- Wake up
- Eat breakfast (hopefully)
- Drive to work
- Sit at a desk
- Eat lunch
- Sit some more
- Eat dinner
- Sit and watch TV
- Go to bed

Notice the trend here? Could it be too much sitting, not enough moving? This is what leads to serious muscle imbalances and so what are we do? We workout in hopes of getting better but the problem worsens due to lack of knowledge.

The key to eliminating back pain is to identify the muscle imbalances that are pulling the spine bones and joints out of place and stretch the tight muscles while strengthening the weak muscles. Most treatment plans offered only address the symptoms and do not address the issue that is causing the symptom, which usually delivers only temporary relief.

Muscle imbalance comes when you have overdeveloped muscles in one area and muscle strain occurs when a muscle or tendon that attaches it to the bone is overextended. This causes the muscle to tear or rip. During my years as a Certified Personal Trainer, I have trained many people and have discovered some wicked facts. Many people who seek professional help are often misdiagnosed and end up following a treatment plan that fails to eliminate the cause of their back pain.

Nearly all the individuals I have worked with who have experienced these issues were able to eliminate their back pain simply by performing a handful of exercises and stretches. They were not your basic exercises or the standard back stretches and stomach exercises most experts recommend. They were specific exercises and stretches prescribed and based on the individual needs.

Simple Overview:

If your core muscles are out of balance in strength verses flexibility perspective, front to back or side to side, you will have at least one postural dysfunction. When your core muscles are out of balance your pelvis will be pulled out of its normal position. Due to the fact that the pelvis is the base of the spine and controls the position and curvature of the spine, your spine will then go into abnormal curvature, which is the root of all back pain - whether it is a pulled back muscle, herniated disk, spinal stenosis, or Si joint!

Flexibility

Flexibility has got to be the most neglected component of physical fitness and probably the most important. Flexibility contributes greatly to your workouts and when properly executed, flexibility will reduce your chances of injury and provide better results. When your muscles are tight, they will pull at your joints, which results in muscle imbalances and injury. I encourage my clients to do dynamic stretching and foam rolling before a workout. Static stretching after each set or after each workout will promote flexibility and elongate the muscles. It helps in recovery as well.

Dynamic Stretching - light jog, squats, jump rope, quad stretches, inchworms – is recommended since this prepares your muscles significantly for a higher level of exercise. Your body should be able to move through a full range of motion to allow blood flow through the muscles. This cannot and should not be done when muscles are cold.

Most injuries happen within the normal range of motion when the muscles are not properly prepared for exercise. This type of stretching is called Static Stretching and can not only cause injury if performed before a workout when your muscles aren't ready for it, but can actually decrease your performance by 10% according to National Academy of Sports Medicine. Static stretching is when you take a muscle to full length and hold it there for a long period of time of thirty seconds or more.

CHAPTER 19

MOTIVATION, MINDSET AND GETTING MENTAL

If I picked one reason people struggle within an exercise program I would have to say it comes from motivation. When I started working out I had no problem with motivation. I guess you have to want it bad enough. I don't like a lot of chitchat during my sessions. I like to get in and get out.

Find what motivates you to get started and once you do you will develop a habit. You may be motivated but just don't know what to do next. Desire and commitment are two different emotions. I recommend you move more and sit less. Refer to Chapter 15 for guidance on where to start an exercise program.

Clean out a closet. Vacuum. Go for a bike ride. Play outside with the kids. Learn how to cook. Make a new recipe. TURN OFF THE TV. When you eat well, you feel good. Nobody is going to do this for you. You must push yourself to get started even if you don't feel like it. That mental stuff is in there. You just have to pull it out and use it. Get focused and go beast mode. NO DISTRACTIONS!

Sometimes I dig really deep and get so mentally focused that I'm the only one in the gym even if it is packed with people. I lift more weight and do twice as many reps as ever before. No, I don't slap myself in the face or scream at the top of my lungs. I just basically go to another place in my mind. My happy PUSH place. Push yourself and just see what happens for 21 days. Most of all you must stay consistent. I can't say this enough. Once you develop that habit it will become a lifestyle. Many fall out before reaching this stage. This is one reason why the statistics on obesity are so outrageous. Don't be that person.

I typically train four to six days a week and incorporate all components of physical fitness: cardio, strength training, balance, power training, flexibility, functional, joint endurance and core.

If lack of motivation does hit, take a day off and see what happens. Try a new workout, swim, walk, do some yoga or pilates, try a new class, get some new sneakers or tights – seek out things that motivate you. Headphones with your favorite music might get you started. What motivates you? That's a question only you can answer. I have two amazing training partners, Brenda and Jana and I look forward to every workout. We have been training together for years constantly changing up our workouts to include every component of physical fitness.

Here are a few tips to help keep you motivated:

1. Set goals. Make it simple and progress to long term goals. Make them realistic and attainable. For example, a short term goal would be walk 3 days a week.
2. Make it fun. Do stuff you enjoy doing. Vary your workout to keep things interesting and fun. It shouldn't have to be boring.
3. Develop a habit. Don't fall back on excuses because you can probably come up with a million. Schedule your workouts as you would any other important activity.
4. Put it on paper. Keep an exercise diary. Record what you did and how you felt. If you didn't feel like working out but did anyway, pat yourself on the back. GOOD JOB!
5. Get a workout partner. Joining forces with people who are after the same thing you are makes it so much easier.
6. Reward yourself. I used to put a dollar in a jar every time I ran 3 miles. At the end of the month I bought a new pair of sneakers or tights.
7. Be flexible. If your simply too busy or tired, take a day or two off. Be easy on yourself if you truly need a break.
8. Listen to your favorite music. Music that really gets you motivated and moving.

CHAPTER 20

MACHINES VS FREE WEIGHTS AND PICKING A PERSONAL TRAINER

Machines

PROS

- Machines, when used properly, are easier for someone who is just beginning an exercise program
- They are less intimidating and help the beginner learn control of certain muscle groups

CONS

- Most machines don't conform to your body anatomically, thereby making them dangerous
- Machines don't work synergistically meaning, most machines only hit one muscle group which means less calories burned

Free Weights

PROS

- They require your core and stabilizers to work synergistically
- They are very versatile
- They burn more calories by hitting more muscle groups
- They work both eccentric and concentrically

- There are more exercises you can do standing up to burn more calories
- They provide you with a bigger variety for more calorie burn

CONS

- Can be potentially dangerous when not used properly
- They can be intimidating
- Proper instructions are needed to execute moves
- If you are not a self starter, you will probably need a personal trainer to learn how to get started with free weights

Picking a Personal Trainer

What exactly are you looking for in a personal trainer? Do you want a trainer that provides motivation, a drill sergeant, cheerleader, maybe someone to instruct you on proper technique and form? Take time to select the trainer that works best with your personality and skill level.

My personal training style is teaching my client what they are doing and why. I'm forever talking about proper form and technique as to get he most out of their workouts. I'm a little too 'drilly' in the fact that I drill proper form into their heads. My specialty is motivation and encouragement to always try for just one more rep. If a client comes back from a week off from the flu, believe me, I won't be pushing them but encouraging them to work at their own pace. To pick up where you left off would be detrimental and possibly set you back even more. There are so many different ways to train. Know what you want and share these details with your Trainer.

No ifs, ands or buts, a personal trainer should be certified and most gyms require this. There is a fine line between making a sound investment in your health and simply throwing money away on something that is not going to work or worse, get you injured. What are your thoughts when you see a Trainer who appears to be out of shape, overweight?

It would be difficult for me to expect more from my clients than I expect from myself. For me personally that puts a little pressure on so to speak. I'm not talking about top form but I believe their body composition should at least be within a healthy range. If you are in the market for a personal trainer, observe the trainers in the gym first to find the right one. Every trainer has his or her own style of teaching and finding the right one may take time but it will be well worth your while! Know their credentials. Do you have physical limitations that would need special attention? Be specific and know what you want and be adamant about it.

Most exercise guidelines are designed specifically for healthy individuals between 18 and 65 years of age. Resistance training among older adults can be very rewarding, highly beneficial and should be recommended as per your doctor. Modifications are definitely in order for the healthy, senior citizen. For example, a push up for a healthy 20-30 year old would obviously look entirely different for a relatively healthy senior citizen who is just starting out. A skilled trainer can provide anyone with a good overall conditioning and flexibility fitness plan. I believe everyone should strive for this no matter what your age is. It's never too late?

Here is a picture of my son, Jeff and I. Now I'm sitting on his shoulders.

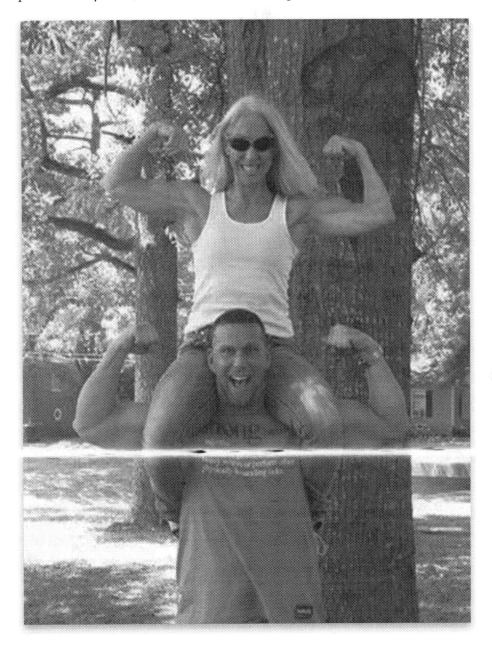

Peace Love & Fitness

~Debbie Crall~

INDEX

strong 25, 44, 46
stronger 3, 20, 28, 29
studio 3, 22, 23, 25, 27
super mom ix, 1, 2, 3, 4
supplement 15, 30, 31, 39, 40
supplements 15, 30, 31, 39, 40
surgery 21, 49
sweat 8
sweating 3
symmetry 8, 10, 14, 28

T

teaching 3, 5, 12, 22, 24, 60
Texarkana 5, 12
Texas 3, 22, 25, 26
toning 48
trainer ix, 9, 10, 22, 24, 43, 49, 55, 59, 60, 61
trainers ix, 9, 10, 22, 24, 43, 49, 55, 59, 60, 61
training xi, 2, 4, 8, 10, 11, 12, 15, 16, 17, 18, 19, 24,
        25, 26, 28, 29, 30, 37, 41, 43, 46, 47, 51, 53, 54,
        58, 60
trans fat 35
trend 39, 55
trends 39, 55
trophies 6
trophy 6, 11, 15

U

Uncle Eric ix, 1

V

vitamins 30

W

warm up 19
warrior xi, 25, 26
water 10, 18, 19, 31, 33, 50
weights 2, 8, 11, 16, 17, 18, 22, 23, 28, 31, 36, 37, 39,
        47, 48, 49, 51, 54, 57, 59, 60
wellness ix
where to begin 43
win 12, 15
winning 6, 8, 9, 10, 15
wins 12, 15
Wisconsin 7, 9, 10
woman 7, 28
women 3, 8, 9, 17, 24, 28, 31, 34
won 6, 8, 9, 10, 11, 60
worked 6, 10, 13, 22, 23, 31, 54, 56
working 1, 2, 3, 11, 17, 22, 23, 25, 32, 40, 44, 54,
        57, 58
working out 1, 2, 3, 11, 17, 23, 25, 32, 54, 57, 58
work out 2
workout 2, 3, 5, 12, 15, 16, 17, 19, 22, 30, 31, 35, 37,
        38, 47, 48, 49, 51, 53, 54, 55, 56, 58, 60
work outs 2
workouts 2, 3, 5, 12, 15, 16, 17, 19, 22, 30, 31, 35, 37,
        38, 47, 48, 49, 51, 53, 54, 55, 56, 58, 60

Y

Yoga 58

Printed in the United States
By Bookmasters